How to Navigate
the Anti-Ageing Maze
And Not Get Lost

How to Navigate the Anti-Ageing Maze And Not Get Lost

*A Novice's Guide
to Cosmetic Injectables*

Dr. Liz Griffin

Library of Congress Control Number:		2012922521
ISBN:	Hardcover	978-1-4797-5759-6
	Softcover	978-1-4797-5758-9
	Ebook	978-1-4797-5760-2

To order additional copies of this book, contact:
Xlibris Corporation
1-800-618-969
www.xlibris.com.au
orders@xlibris.com.au
502595

CONTENTS

CREDITS

1. Lady Lisa on page 12—Photographed by Sandy Powers. URL Source: *http://twistedsifter.com/2010/11/picture-of-the-day-every-picture-tells-a-story-nov-30-2010/*

2. Baby Boy on Page 11: *http://t1.thpservices.com/fotos/thum4/018/241/fnc-42-27523916.jpg*

3. Old lady on page 23: *http://www.bluesalley.net/Fans/old_lady.jpg*

OVERVIEW

I have worked in anti-ageing medical skin care in Sydney Australia since 1985. I have also worked in skin cancer clinics in city. Sydney is blessed with a long Summer and a short Winter. It is also blessed with sunshine all through the year.

We complain if it rains or if the sun is clouded over. Our Winter is not like winter in Europe. We might have a grey overcast day once in a while but mainly the sun shines and the sky is bright blue. If you can get out of the cold wind it is perfectly possible to sit in a sunny spot and sun bake in winter, and we do. There are many beaches in Sydney, all easily accessible and close to the city.

This creates an environment where good, healthy, youthful skin is the exception not the norm. The first impression that the English and other Northern Europeans have of us is that the women look so old. When sun damaged skin is the norm it is difficult to persuade people to try and improve their skin. Tans are no longer fashionable as fashionable as they were, and tanning beds will soon be illegal in this country. Spray tanning is the acceptable alternative and is becoming very common. Perhaps the nation's skin will improve.

One thing that may bring us back to good skin is the interest in anti—ageing treatments, mainly injectable products.

If we concede that most of our wrinkles are caused by sun damage and that sun exposure is bad for us, it is surprising the number of clients who are obsessed with removing all their wrinkles but have no interest in trying to reverse the sun damage that caused them.

Perhaps we need to wait for the next sun protected generation to grow up. Our children are perhaps the best protected anywhere. Parents protect their young children obsessively. Child care centres have shade cloth over the play areas. School children cannot go out to play if they don't have their hat. Children are anointed with sunscreen every day. Sunscreen is provided at worksites. Labourers are not permitted to work with their shirts off. But the incidence of malignant melanoma in young people is going up.

Somewhere between childhood and adulthood we are still losing the battle.

The fashion for tans has abated a little and the fashion for no lines has increased a lot. The number of those seeking treatment for their lines has gone up in both males and females. Women are leading the charge and their men are following, albeit a little reluctantly.

Perhaps once we have their lines under control then we can improve the skins as well.

Our citizens are aware of skin cancer, but they are not worried about it because it is so common. Either everyone has it or knows someone who does. Older people go to skin cancer clinics three to six monthly to have liquid nitrogen sprayed on patches of precancerous skin. They all call it skin cancer, but it isn't, not yet. It is so common people think it's normal to have patches of red scaly skin on the face, neck and hands. Their main complaint is that liquid nitrogen hurts and causes scabs on the area of treatment for ten days.

While Australians are complaisant about precancerous skin disease, they are very concerned about malignant melanoma but less so about basal cell carcinomas and squamous cell carcinomas, again because they see these as normal. However once they or someone close to them develops a basal cell carcinoma that requires the nose and half the face to be excised and then reconstructed they are shocked. I think it comes back to the overall belief that red, scaly skin is skin cancer and not a warning. They are so used to having all their precancerous spots treated every year that they forget that skin cancer itself is more serious.

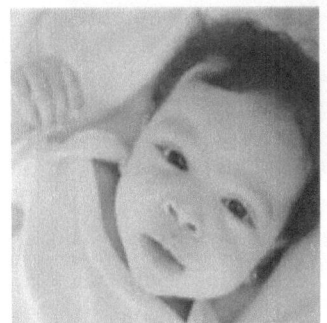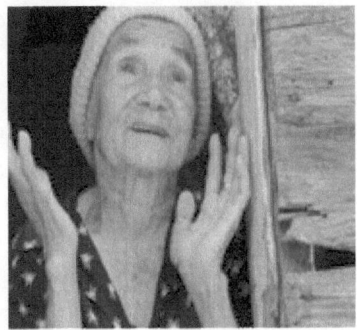

The baby's skin and the old lady's skin started out the same. What happened to make that change?

We know that some are genetically blessed and keep their good skins into old age but most of us do not. We know the cause of the change—the sun and poor diet, plus cigarettes. Because we know the cause we are now given the choice as to which type of skin we want to have, and some choose the sun damaged one. The baby's is clear and translucent, even in tone, perfect in texture. The old woman's is dull and lifeless, opaque, irregularly pigmented and wrinkled.

In the absence of the desire for good skin clinicians can only treat as requested—but we keep trying.

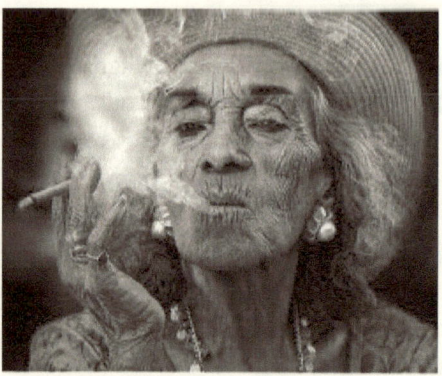

This woman has very good bone structure. Her proportions are good. Do you get the feeling that her lifestyle has had something to do with her ageing?

Whatever I can do I can't make sun exposure non damaging and I can't stop the damaging effect of smoking and or poor diet.

People come to me and ask for the same things over and over. They don't like the frown line, their crow's feet and their forehead lines. Most people are unaware of what can be treated and how it can best be done.

So this is a guide for the client who wants to know more. Very few people are aware of what can and cannot be achieved to improve appearance without surgery. Their knowledge is limited to the things they have experienced. Most are very confused by the number of different treatment methods available and advertised. Everyone in business pushes their own type of treatment whether it be the beautician who has a microdermabrasion machine or the plastic surgeon who knows all about surgery. Each thinks his own is the way to go. How is the lay person to understand, let alone chose sensibly?

My expertise is in non-surgical facial rejuvenation so I will not comment on surgical options. Let someone else do that.

I do not believe that it is practical nor desirable for an eighty year old woman to try to look like a twenty year old.

With surgery it might be possible if the skin quality were good and her general health excellent, but just consider hands, feet, toes, arms . . . . If the skin quality were poor and paper thin then healing would be a major concern. She would be in hospital for months.

In any case how many people would want to have such extreme surgery? How many eighty year olds would survive the surgery? Facial rejuvenation is not about taking very old people and trying to make them look very young. It is about maintaining a mature person's appearance over the long term.

It is certainly possible to maintain an adult at an indeterminate age without making such person look weird—the hated "other species look". It is however a matter of judgement as to how much should be done.

This judgement tends to become unreliable in some clients and some doctors once they become used to their new look. They in fact become addicted to their new look and want more. It is a good idea to listen to an honest judgement from your doctor over whether or not to have more filler, more muscle relaxants but remember the doctor is not a disinterested party in this because his profit is affected by how much you have. I have seen clients have too much and regretfully have to say that profit blurred the doctor's judgement.

For most people embarking on this road their first priority is not to be noticed and ridiculed by their friends and family. If you see that the person approaching you with the needle in hand looks over done then I suggest you leave and go elsewhere. This sort of rejuvenation should not be obvious unless you live in a community where looking "plastic" is the norm.

There are certain areas in this city where the big lip and frozen face look are common. Thankfully it is not widespread. If you live in an area where it is common then you will not be as afraid as the majority are here.

Even if you live in a society that embraces the overdone look it is a good idea to seek out someone whose clients come out looking normal. Good rejuvenation work is not visible!

A person's age is relevant when deciding what treatments are suitable, what is over kill and what is too little. Young women need very little to make them look great, particularly if they have worn sunscreen religiously from childhood and their skin is good. Unfortunately some twenty five year olds have excessive sun damage and they are regular clients for anti-wrinkle injections.

We still see some who were brought up on the beach, used olive oil and lemon juice to increase their tan and it is no surprise that they show visible signs of ageing greater than their better protected peers. Those who live outside cities and closer to the equator are less likely to protect their skins. This is either through lack of knowledge or lack of concern.

We know that most facial ageing is caused by exposure to sunlight. There is of course a genetic component to skin ageing but the vast amount of damage seen is due to sun exposure.

A recent survey done in the UK shows an incidence of sun related precancerous lesions on the face to be 2—4% of males. In Australia the incidence is 55% in males and 39% in women. If we add to that the incidence of sun damage other than precancerous problems we would find it to be almost universal. Sun damage causes wrinkling of the skin, irregular pigmentation, enlarged pores and enlarged veins.

Young women under the age of thirty are usually concerned about movement related lines around the eyes (crow's feet), frown lines and horizontal lines. For most of them the lines are present only on movement. Some do have the lines present at rest and this indicates more severe sun damage.

It is appropriate to treat those clients with lines present at rest with injections of muscle relaxants.

At present there is a movement towards preventing any lines at all. Young women without lines at rest want treatment to stop those lines developing and want to use muscle relaxants to do it. Will this work long term for them? I think there is a better chance is they use good sun protection and skin repair products.

When I say muscle relaxants I mean either Botox or Dysport. These are the two botulinum toxin products licenced for use in Australia at present. Another is about to hit our shores and there are other brands available in America and Europe. These products are essentially the same. There are minor differences but not much.

Treatment of crow's feet, frown lines and horizontal forehead lines is a very simple treatment. It takes about five minutes and leaves minimal evidence that anything has been done. Occasionally bruising occurs and that is usually at the outer corner of the eye.

Older women have other concerns. Certainly they need to wear their sunscreen and will probably need muscle relaxant injections but they will also need to deal with the fact that we lose the fat pads in the face as we age and that bone thinning is not restricted to the spine and the long bones. We also lose bone thickness in facial bones particularly the mandible.

The neck becomes a focus of concern after the age of forty and hands after fifty. For those who have not paid attention to their skin sun damage becomes much more obvious. The production of collagen is much decreased after age thirty and skin loses its lovely youthful glow.

We have all been sold "hope in a jar." In fact I recently was presented with a cosmetic that was called exactly that. It had no ingredient list, no instructions for use and probably was not in any way active. It had been bought on the internet and promised great results. It did not seem to have given any improvement to the person who bought it. But she didn't think she had been cheated. She didn't expect it to work although it came with lots of endorsements.

The cosmetics industry is huge. To be allowed to be sold as a cosmetic in this country the product must not cause any change in the body, including the skin—otherwise it has to be classified as a drug. Basically, to be sold here as a cosmetic it has to be guaranteed not to do anything!

When you consider that mainstream companies spend very little on the ingredients in their bottles and jars and much more on the containers and bottles and much, much more on advertising it should not come as a surprise that most of these products do not work. There are products that do work and they are those available from doctor's offices and some high end day spas. There are a few that are readily available but by and large those easily available don't work.

Older women definitely need sun damage treatment but they are often frightened by the things we suggest—facial peeling, laser treatment, platelet rich plasma injection. Their comfort zone does not extend past the pot of inactive cream so we have to start very slowly. They are open to the suggestion of injection of dermal fillers.

The areas of the face that require filling as time goes on are the following

- The temples—very few people notice this themselves but loss of fat in the temples is very ageing.

- The tear troughs—this is one of the first areas to go creating a depression and darkness under the eye and onto the cheek.

- The cheekbone. This area loses fat more in some people than others. Lack of fat in the apple of the cheek causes extreme flatness of the mid face and a very aged look.

- The area under the cheekbone—this sculpted look is great when young but causes gauntness when older. In the seventies in Paris it was a fad to remove these fat pads through the inside of the mouth giving the fashion model look instantly. I am sure that these women are now looking for the cheek to be filled out again.

- Marionette lines at the corner of the mouth—these give the owner an unhappy look and are associated with down turning of the angles of the mouth.

- Lip lines and thin lips—top lip lines increase as the bone resorbtion in the maxilla increases. It is not specifically caused by smoking although smoker's have a worse problem associated with the number of free radicles they pump into their bodies. Lower lip lines occur as well. The lips themselves lose volume and become creased and thin.

- The jawline and jowls—this is the one thing that says across the room, this woman is on the wrong side of forty.

In Australia we have converted to large scale filling. We like to use as much as possible to give the patient a result comparable to a face lift. Naturally this is limited by the patient's funds. The trend world wide is for less facial surgery i.e the number of face lifts being done has gone down everywhere.

Facial filling is a much more attractive idea. It is safer. There is minimal downtime. There is much less pain. There is no need for hospitalisation. The result is almost instantaneous. The results can be comparable if large volumes are used. By this I mean 10-12 mls of filler in one or two sessions.

The filler products we use most commonly are made of hyaluronic acid and can be removed. Hyaluronic acid is normal component of skin. Its function is to hold water in the skin. The injectable form performs the same function. It holds water in the gel until the gel is destroyed. The length of time the gel lasts varies depending on the product.

The benefit of hyaluronic acid fillers is that they can be removed easily by injection of an enzyme that dissolves the product. This hurts at the time but it is very effective and is certainly better than having to cut out the problem.

There are other fillers that cannot be dissolved. These include polylactic acid (sculptra), Aquamid, and Calcium hydroxyapetite (Radiesse). There are more brands offered in Europe and USA but these are the only ones offered here.

Sulptra and Radiesse are implants that rely on the body's ability to produce connective tissue (collagen) in response to the injection. The connective tissue actually replaces the product and produces a good long lasting result.

There are complications associated with Sculptra that come from the way it works. Overgrowth of connective tissue can occur and results in lumps deep to and in the skin. These can be difficult to treat. In my practice I have never seen such a complication from Sculptra but it does exist. Most of the explanations for this relate to poor mixing of the product (it does not come premixed) and poor injection technique. Sometimes statistics are statistics and we experience all our complications in one short period and sometimes they are spread out. So probably my bad results are coming next year, or the year after. I do like this product particularly for patients with large volume loss because it is not as expensive as other large volume fillers and allows the patient to have larger amounts.

Because we have an obligation to tell our patients the relative benefits and potential complications of the treatment we suggest then the incidence of granulomas (skin lumps) has to be disclosed. The incidence is fifteen times the incidence with hyaluronic acid. Most patients opt for the safer product.

Radiesse works in the same way by encouraging an increase in connective tissue. So far there have not been reports of lumps resulting from its use. It has its good points but is very unforgiving and has a tendency to look hard.

Aquamid is a permanent filler. That is it cannot be removed except by surgery. For most patients this is the thing they want—permanence. As we age we will also age around a permanent implant so the permanence is not as relevant as one would think. As the tissue sags around the implant more needs to be injected. Some people are very happy with its use in their lips but others are not happy with the shape or the size and they are stuck with it. There have been cases of complications from Aquamid that were very difficult to manage. These were mainly infection in the implant itself or incorrect placement. Anything that is placed inside the body as a permanent implant is a risk for infection. This is why orthopaedic surgeons are so concerned about operating on a patient with any infection anywhere. Patients are refused surgery on the booked date for this reason.

Manufacturers of other fillers always state that their product should not be used over a permanent filler because they do not want their product embroiled in a problem of not their own making. Patients who are unhappy because they have developed an unpleasant side effect have a tendency to sue the doctor and the product manufacturer. Most lawyers will add anyone who could possibly be involved in the poor outcome to the law suit. So the innocent product can be tainted by the guilty one. Most doctors will not inject over a permanent implant with a semi-permanent filler for the same reason.

Hyaluronic acid fillers can result in lumps but because the products can be dissolved they are not such a treatment problem

Some patients say that they want to have only one procedure done in their life. They want to wait till it's really bad and then have a definitive procedure that should last until their death. I cannot identify with this idea although I have heard it many times. It does not sit well with the more common refrain of "I don't want anyone to know." To me it is like saying I won't buy new clothes until these fall off me and I'm wearing rags. Naturally a major intervention such as a face lift is very obvious in an older patient. They go from very lax skin to very taut skin in a week or two and everybody notices. Perhaps they are too well mannered to say anything but they certainly notice.

Why would anyone wait so long to do anything? Doesn't it make more sense to keep up with the deterioration on a regular basis so that clients remain a certain indeterminate age for ever?

If large volume filling is done sufficiently well, patients should need a top up every year but never a mega fill again. Naturally patients will continue to need muscle relaxants regularly and to continue with good skin care.

Very saggy necks will still need surgery, but for less sagging there are other techniques.

Necks can be treated with fillers and muscle relaxants. Filler treatment in the neck is directed at repairing the skin and tightening it rather than filling defects. Muscle relaxants in the neck are used to contour the jawline.

Thermage is also a suitable treatment for sagging necks. Clients must not have too much sagging for this to be effective. Thermage and Ulthera are radio frequency treatments. They tighten the skin by heating it and changing the type of collagen present in the skin.

DESIRED SHAPES AND RATIOS

Not everyone is born beautiful, but most are born with an acceptable level of good looks. When we can find someone born without beauty but who can be made beautiful by a few well—placed filler injections it would be a crime not to do it!

We perceive beauty the same way across all ethnic groups.

Our preferred facial shape is oval. We like symmetry and the more symmetrical a face is the more beautiful we perceive it to be.

We like the face to be divided equally horizontally into three zones of roughly similar length, and vertically into five zones.

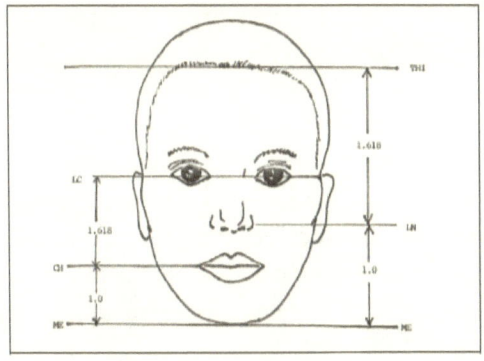

Vertical Proportion

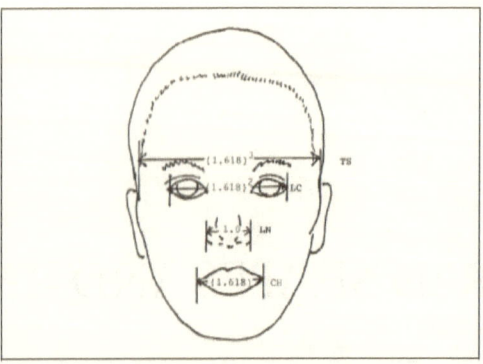

Transverse Proportion

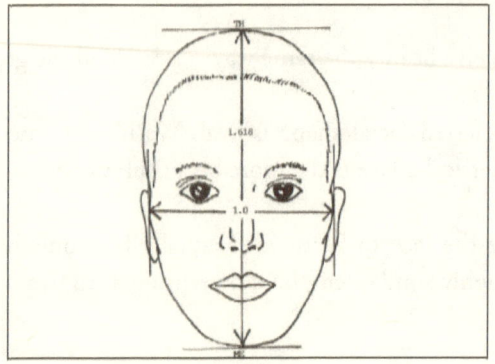

External Proportion

This gives us a very mathematical measurement of beauty and appeals to the scientist. Whilst this may not interest you, you will all call the same mathematical relationships of elements of the face beautiful. Most of the measurable ratios in the face should be related to *phi*. The closer we can bring a client's face to the correct ratio the more beautiful she will be.

Many attempts have been made to develop a reproducible system of ratios that physicians can work from to create beautiful and harmonious faces. Marquardt's mask is one of these systems. All the facial measurements are said to be able to be related to the golden ratio *phi*. It is tempting to believe that mathematically derived systems can give us the perfect blue print for beauty but they have all been challenged one way or another. For some, beauty exists in the unusual rather than the predicted, for the others we must still rely on approximations to the ratios.

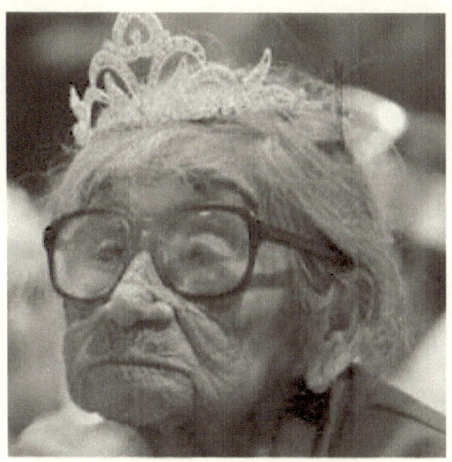

This lady has obvious fat loss in her cheeks but fixing that will not improve her appearance much. The proportions of her face are abnormal with her chin being too short. With age the nasal tip drops and the chin turns upward making the face shorter. Lots of fillers in combination with fixing the chin proportion would make this lady more attractive.

The purpose of these analyses is to help the physician move a patient closer towards these ideals and therefore make her more beautiful. There is no great point in trying to make someone look ordinary if you can make them look beautiful. Obviously there are people who will never be model beautiful but there are many who could be much more attractive by making the eyebrow higher, lengthening a chin, widening the cheekbones and enlarging the mouth, slimming the jawline and recontouring the cheeks. A good cosmetic physician will be interested in making these changes as well as simply removing facial lines.

Over the next pages I want to look at individual problems and show you how they are best treated

FOREHEAD PROBLEMS

The commonest request a cosmetic physician will hear is, "fix my frown line".

This is usually done with muscle relaxants like Botox or Dysport that are injected into the muscles responsible for the specific problem.

Frown lines are the vertical lines that occur above the root of the nose, across the eyebrow, and across the top of the nose. Patients think that everyone perceives them as cranky when they are not.

Some patients have very strong muscles in this area and develop very deep vertical lines. Others have a series of vertical lines going out towards the temple, while others pull down very strongly across the top of the nose creating a deep horizontal line. Still others have little movement towards the nose but pull their eyebrows down to frown. Others pull their eyebrows together and their foreheads up resulting in an upside down U.

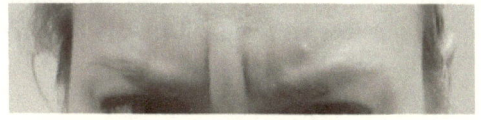

This is an example of very strong muscles, with a lot of downward pull by circular muscle of the eye and an extension of the frown muscles to the mid eyebrow.

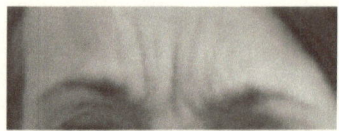

This woman has less strong muscles but she has multiple muscle attachments along the inner brow. Different people need different injection points.

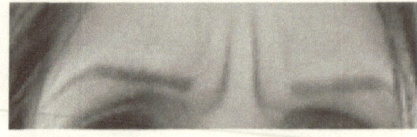

This lady has no lateral insertion points of her frown muscles (the corrugators)but she has a very strong set of muscles

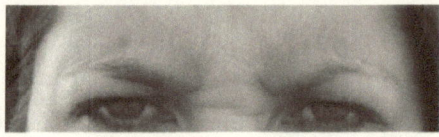

The most prominent muscle activity in this lady when she frowns, is that she pulls the centre of her forehead down towards her nose, creating a horizontal line.

Each of these types of frown needs different placement of the injections. So on your first visit you will always be asked to frown a few times.

Muscle relaxants last three to four months. If too little has been injected it won't last as long. After you have been treated regularly for about a year your muscles will become smaller and your treatment is likely to last longer—maybe even five or six months. Not everyone finds this but some do.

Most doctors don't like to use fillers in this area. Most will use a muscle relaxant and then recall the patient to see how good the result is. If the line is still very visible then you will be offered a filler as well. You will usually be reassessed at two weeks because it takes that long to get the full benefit of the muscle relaxant treatment.

Combination treatment like this lasts up to nine months and will be necessary for those who have deep sharp frown lines. This is probably about one in fifty people treated. Most will get away with simple muscle relaxants.

The reason that doctors don't like injecting fillers in this area is that the vascular supply to the area can be compromised by incorrect filler placement. This is not a common complication and the doctor will be well equipped to handle it should it occur.

HORIZONTAL FOREHEAD LINES

These lines come about because of constant muscular activity involved in raising the eyebrows. This is a natural part of the greeting process in humans. Think of it next time you see someone you know in the street. Your eyebrows will go up as you recognise them. Some people do this more than others and consequently develop deeper lines.

And we raise our eyebrows when surprised and shocked.

The other reason we raise our eyebrows is to lift the eyelids. As people age their eyebrows drift lower thus increasing the sagginess of the upper eyelids. People whose eyelids are sagging will try to lift them all the time. Every time we look in a mirror we do it. We all look better when we lift our eyebrows a little. Also it seems to be impossible to put on mascara and not raise the eyebrows.

Horizontal forehead lines are best treated by muscle relaxants. Fillers can be used but may leave visible lumps. The difficulty when treating horizontal forehead lines with muscle relaxant is that overtreatment can cause the brows to drop. This is not a desirable effect, so often a compromise must be reached.

A drop of even 1 mm is detectable by the patient and makes them feel very heavy lidded. Anything more than this will need to be treated.

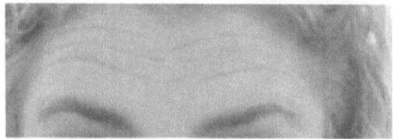

These horizontal lines will never be completely removed by muscle relaxant injections. They have been there too long and are too deep. They will be reduced in depth and that may be all the client wants.

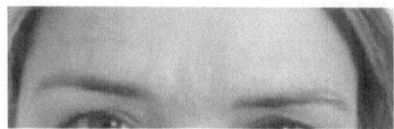

Note the drooping of the eyelid skin before treatment. This patient would look very tired if her brows fell. It might be wise to ignore the forehead lines.

Several injection patterns can be used depending on the individual musculature. Injecting in the main belly of the muscle is more likely to cause brow drop. Patients who have a very short forehead are also at higher risk of dropping of the brow. Those with a very short forehead should only be injected with muscle relaxants high on the forehead or with reduced amounts of relaxant.

Some people develop a very sharp inverted V in their eyebrows from thoughtless placement of the injections. This is referred to as "Spocking" after Mr Spock from Start Trek. Usually this can be predicted and avoided. If it occurs it should respond to more correctly targeted treatment. There are some people who specifically request this result. Personally I think it looks bizarre.

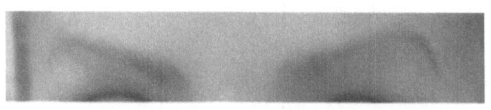

Our eyes are one of the primary focus areas of the face. Speaking to people face to face we concentrate on the eyes, so they are very important. If I can make a client's eyes look more open I think I have done a good treatment because it removes some of the tiredness that we all complain of.

Most people are concerned with their crow's feet but I think that brow placement and eye openness is more important and creates more impact.

Crow's feet come in all lengths. Some are just small laugh lines at the side of the eye, others are so long that they extend to half way down the cheek and open up in a fan from above the eye to well below. Most are restricted to the area just adjacent to the outside of the eye.

These can be treated by placing tiny injections of muscle relaxant in three or four places at the side of the eye. This will remove most lines. It looks odd if the lateral crow's feet are completely removed and a long under eye line is allowed to remain. It should be stopped at the outer edge of the eye.

The lines under the eye should not be treated with relaxants because the muscles that control the tension under the eye will be weakened and fat that exists normally under the eye will protrude creating a bulge or bag under the eye. This will remain until the effect wears off about twelve weeks later. Some doctors are practising what they call "meso Botox". This refers to the use of highly diluted muscle relaxant injected in all areas and comes from the term Mesotherapy. It can be used under the eye but will not last long.

Injections should not be placed closer than one cm to the bony rim of the orbit. This is easily felt with the injector's finger. Injections placed too close to the orbit can cause two problems. One, the relaxant may drift into the muscles that control the movement of the eye (a very rare complication), causing double vision, or two, the skin under the eye may bunch up on movement.

Trying to remove long, low crow's feet by chasing them down the cheek can cause a problem if the muscle controlling smiling (zygomaticus) is injected. This cannot be corrected and will need to wear off. Some crow's feet should simply be left there.

When muscle relaxants are not useful there are other treatments that are. The area under the eye is one such area. The treatment varies depending on whether the client has had cosmetic eye surgery or not. Those who have had surgery will usually end up hollow under the eyes. They need filling between the cheek and the eye. This needs to be done carefully and finely. The last thing that will help the client is too much filler under the eye. Those who have not had surgery need filling lower down just between the hollow and the cheek. A blunt tipped cannula is essential here otherwise bruising will be severe.

Another way of treating this area is to use laser ablation either full or partial. This will tighten the skin and remove lines but will not give a perfect result. The hollowing will still remain although it will be obscured by swelling from the laser treatment for some time. It will eventually need to be treated. Both treatments can be used one after the other but not together. It is sensible to do only what needs to be done and wait after each treatment.

EYEBROWS

Eyebrows frame the eyes and are very important in appearance of the face. Eyebrows too high and people think you saw a ghost. Eyebrows too low and they perceive an aged appearance. Please note this applies mainly to women. It is a masculine characteristic to have a narrow distance between the eyebrows and the eyes and increasing that distance imparts a feminine look.

The area where treatment can make the greatest impact is the eyebrow. The brow can be naturally straight and flat and look great, but the most commonly preferred type is the high arched brow that flares at the side. This is the shape you see in all the eye makeup advertisements.

This can be achieved for most people by injecting the area under the brow with a muscle relaxant. This stops the pull down effect caused by the circular muscle around the eye. The injections are placed to weaken this muscle at the upper outer half of the eyebrow and at the side of the eye. This muscle (orbicularis oculi) performs a tug of war with the muscle that raises the eyebrows (frontalis). To have the effect you want movement must be present before treatment. In other words if you can't raise your eyebrow in the desired area we cannot give you that movement. Most people can raise the brow 3-10 mm at the outer edge. This can make a major improvement to the appearance of the eyes.

Some people look better if the inner part of the eyebrow is raised or the whole eyebrow. If the inner part of the eyebrow is too low people look cross and owlish. This can occur as a side effect of injecting muscle relaxant to remove the frown lines. Thankfully this can be corrected quite easily by injecting a small muscle just under the inner end of the brow (levator supercilii).

Raising the brow has the added effect of decreasing the sagginess of the upper eyelid skin. To get the best effect the circular muscle around eye must be relaxed at the outer corner as well. This will also decrease the crow's feet a little bit.

CROW'S FEET

This again is an area where treatment is often requested. Most clinicians treat this area with muscle relaxants although some will use a very low strength filler in the area. Treatment of the cheekbone area with fillers will result in improvement in crow's feet further from the eye.

The placement of injections around the eyes is dictated by where the lines are in motion. You will probably be asked to smile. This doesn't mean screw your eyes up tight! Everyone is going to have some lines around the eyes when they screw their eyes up tight. Even children will. Just smile naturally when asked.

The lines that radiate from the corner of the eye are easily treated with a few well—placed injections of relaxant. Bruises can occur in this area but if the injector is careful they are rare. It is impossible to say that it will never happen because it does sometimes. There are many small blood vessels in this area and sometimes one will be hit with a needle and cause bruising.

Like all bruises it will take ten days to go away.

Bruises are not the worst thing that can happen. Patients want all the lines to go away and often request injections that would be too close to the eye or in an area that just shouldn't be injected.

It is not a good idea to inject past the outer corner of the eye underneath the eye because it will weaken the muscles there. That can result in a bag appearing under the eye. Trying to chase lines down the cheek from the eye too far can result in a problem with the muscles of the mouth. Accept it, there will still be some fine lines. Fillers used to increase the volume of the cheek can be helpful here. Naturally you will get added benefits from that.

Under eye lines can be treated quite well in other ways. Fraxel laser treatment will remove them but will probably need to be done several times. Thermage will tighten the skin and remove the lines as well. Injectables are not the only tool in the tool box.

The newer cosmesceutical preparations are also very effective. If you don't believe you can get results from a cream then you haven't been using the right cream. Most of these newer creams take six months of continual application to decrease eye lines but they do work. Before and after photos are very telling.

It is probably still inevitable that surgery will become necessary at some stage but we can certainly put it off for a long time. When surgery (blepharoplasty) is performed on the eyelids skin and fat is removed from the upper and lower eyelid. This removes sag and improves the bags. Such surgery lasts a long time and gives good results but until it is necessary leave it alone. Laser surgery offers a quicker recovery and less bruising but that is all. The technique is slightly different as the lower lid incision is inside the lid rather than through the skin. The incision on the upper lid is the same. Irrespective of the type of surgery the eyelids will be healed in seven to ten days with a scalpel and five to seven days if a laser is used.

Scarring from blepharoplasty is usually minor. It heals well and the scars when well placed are almost invisible.

TEMPLES

This is an area very few people look at. As we age the fat pads in the temple area become less and less and a depression appears. This depression can be quite deep.

It is one of the subliminal clues in a face that tell us a person is old. If you look at old and very unwell people this depression is highly visible. Some of us hide it behind a hair style not even realising it's there. Most don't see it until it is pointed out. When it is corrected no one notices specifically but the face will look younger and healthier just from this one intervention.

There are two techniques for treating this area with fillers. One involves injecting fillers superficially just under the skin. The other requires the injection to be done deeper. I prefer the latter because it will never show and because a very long lasting filler can be used giving a long lasting result.

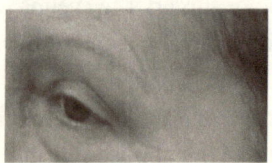

The temples of this woman are very indented and give her an old appearance. Correction would make her look much younger.

CHEEKBONES

We all admire high well defined cheekbones but we don't all have them. With the introduction of long lasting fillers it is possible to give a patient the cheek bones she has always wanted without surgery. Some patients use this type of treatment to significantly improve their looks or for repair after injury. The introduction of Sub Q made by Q-med and Voluma distributed by Allergan gives us a product that will last one to two years without significant side effects. Add to this the introduction of Pix'l cannulae and we have a treatment that will last a long time and not cause much bruising and discomfort and will significantly improve the appearance of the face. Because increasing the volume of the cheeks and cheekbones lifts the skin and replaces lost fat pads this can make patients look much younger. It really can be the much advertised "face lift in your lunch time".

The alternative is a surgical cheekbone implant. These have been used in association with a surgical facelift and also alone to contour the cheek. When used with a facelift they are essentially being used to increase the mid-face volume. This is what we are doing with long lasting injectables with a lot less down time. In my opinion surgical implants look too hard and too big and not natural. I much prefer to see cheekbones augmented with dermal fillers. They are softer feeling and softer looking. They are easily inserted and easily removed. It is necessary to top up the product one to two yearly but no hospital visit or anaesthesia is needed. Also there is minimal recovery time. Which would you choose?

We use these products in anti-ageing medicine because we lose fat pads in the face with age. The most commonly lost fat pads are those in the mid face. This leads to drooping of the facial skin and slackness of the jaw. If we think of the facial skin as a table cloth laid on a base of muscle, fat and bone and consider that all these elements shrink or disappear with age, then it will come as no surprise that the tablecloth is drooping, looking too big for the base.

We can take the skin back, tighten the muscles, cut off the excess skin and then replace the skin and stitch it back on. This is the traditional face lift. Or we can increase the bulk of the base. When we consider that face lifts are done in operating theatres, take approximately five hours to do, have a significant incidence of heamatoma formation requiring a return to theatre, and a long recovery period, deep facial filling is an attractive treatment as it can be done through a needle and has very little side effect or downtime.

This is a very effective treatment provided enough filler is used and can take the place of a face lift unless there is a lot of neck looseness. Some patients have this type of treatment following a face lift as they find that their facial contours are not as pretty as they could be particularly in front of the ear and in the cheek. If we consider the concept of fat loss and bone loss a face lift is going to tighten the skin over a smaller skeleton and less padding. It is not going to return youth to the face.

To treat the cheek and cheekbone area a small area of skin is injected with local anaesthetic and a tiny incision is made with a needle. The filler is introduced through here via a long blunt needle (cannula). The cannula has a rounded tip and will not go through blood vessels. Before the introduction of cannulae we used sharp tipped needles. The needles caused a lot of bruising because they went straight through veins. Cannulae will never cause as much bleeding as a sharp needle but bruising is still possible although it is rare. Clients on clopidogrel should not have these treatments.

Clients on Warfarin will bruise and perhaps should not have dermal fillers. They will be fine with muscle relaxants and superficial fillers but they will bruise. Asprin, ginko biloba and fish oils should also be avoided for ten days before treatment.

The product will be introduced via the cannula in a fan like distribution so that the cheek can be filled throughout a distance of approximately six to ten centremetres. Sometimes a number of entry points will be required. What is really astonishing about this technique is that there is very little pain. Usually patients feel the initial local anaesthetic point and just some weird feelings of pushing and pulling. Some patients find that they hear the product going in and making a crackling sound. These products contain local anaesthetic so the anaesthesia increases as the treatment proceeds.

To get the best result possible we use a large amount of filler for the first treatment and top that up once a year thereafter. The initial treatment will be expensive but the maintenance will not. What you get is continued improvement that looks natural and can be tailored to changes as they occur.

Most patients will be back at work the following day with the only evidence of their procedure being that they look great and have a couple of tiny steri-strips on the cheek.

The area of treatment can be tender for the following few days. Asprin should be avoided. Panadol should be used if necessary. If you compare this with a face lift which requires a week in hospital or being looked after, potential haematomas, a general anaesthetic and lots of stitches it should be easy to understand why filler procedures are increasing in popularity. These operations are also costly. Most surgeons charge ten to twenty thousand dollars. The hospital bill will not be rebateable under insurance and can run into thousands of dollars as well. It is not a very attractive proposition. It is unlikely that you will be back at work following a face lift for at least two weeks. This is another cost that should be factored in.

The most significant side effect encountered so far with deep injection of long lasting fillers is infection in the treated areas. This is not common but it has occurred enough for most doctors to be at least contemplating giving the patient a single large dose of oral antibiotic at the time of treatment.

It is my practice to give patients 1gm of Amoxycillin or Cephalexin at the time of treatment and to postpone treatment of patients who have a pre-existing infection.

Treatment of the infection is not difficult, usually requiring three weeks of antibiotic treatment. In some cases the product has to be dissolved as well. This will require injection of an enzyme called hylase. This product is equally as expensive as the filler itself. It removes the hyaluronic acid implant almost instantaneously.

I tried to show you changes on the faces of some well-known people but unfortunately with litigation being what it is I'll illustrate all my facial changes over the years instead.

Let's start with my First Communion photo, aged 7.

As you can see I have a very rounded oval face. My cheeks are very full and my eyes are very prominent.

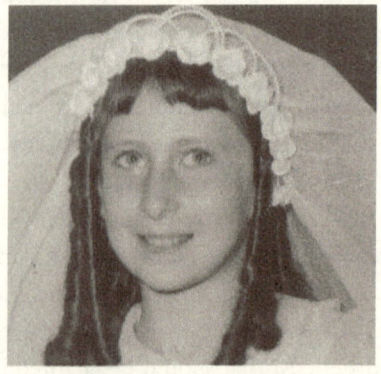

Rag curls must have been fashionable and nylon reigned supreme. I have no wrinkles and good clear skin.

This next one was taken when I was about seventeen, living in a convent boarding school where we used to have to cut each other's hair. Luckily this time I had a professional hair-cut. Not much has changed since the previous photo, although I have a few freckles and my face is not quite as round.

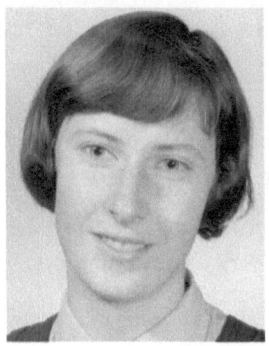

The next one is a little later and is here purely so you don't wonder why my nose looks different as I age.

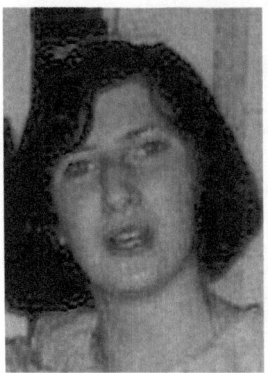

This was taken the evening of the day my nose was broken by a softball. You can see it is swollen and somewhat askew.

This next photo was taken when I was about 36.

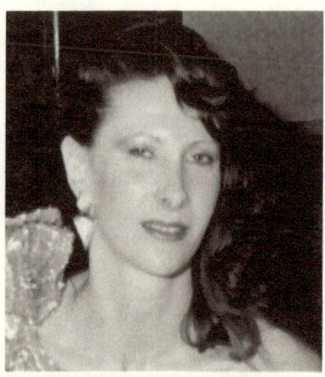

You can see the beginning of a depression under the eyes and a further slimming of the lower face making the cheekbones more prominent. You will note that I had my nose fixed, but it left an unsightly lump on the right side of the tip, which is not a good result.

This next one is about ten years later. You can see that the tip of my nose has been fixed,(I still have a crooked nose). The depressions under the eyes are deeper and the face has continued to slim in the cheeks.

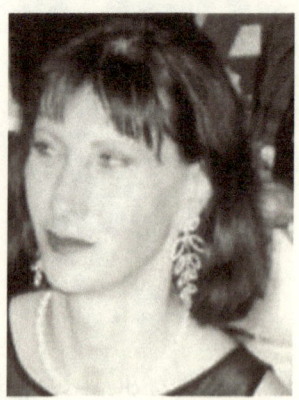

Now I am going to treat you to an amateur photo of me taken in my office by the receptionist. I am now 63 and things have changed!

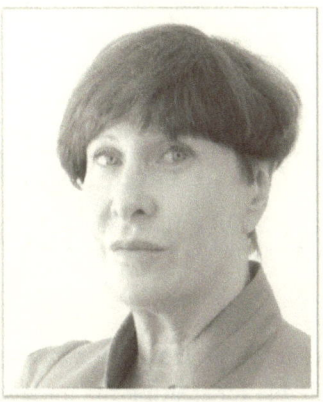

This isn't a very good photograph but you can easily see the ageing changes. I have lost a lot of fat directly under my eyes and in my upper cheeks. My neck needs the muscular bands relaxed and possibly some laser treatment to the skin to tighten it up a little. The naso-labial folds are prominent, reflecting fat loss in the cheek and the jawline is no longer crispThere is also a little hooding over the right eye.

It's time for me to go and visit a friend of mine and get a little work done! Just a little, because I'm not young anymore and nothing I do will make me look young. However I can still look attractive and real.

TEAR TROUGHS
AND UNDER EYE HOLLOWS

Eye bags and hollows are very ageing. We discussed earlier that Botox /Dysport are not suitable for treating the under eye area. Fillers can be used to improve this area if used appropriately.

The dent that occurs under the eye starting near the nose and running down outwards to the cheek is called the tear trough. For some it is a very deep dent and makes them look tired even when they are not. This can be filled with a medium strength dermal filler with a good result.

Poor results occur if too much filler is put there or if it is placed too superficially. Too much filler over corrects and makes the problem worse. Too superficial placement causes swelling, oedema and sometimes visible product. These problems will all go away but can take time. If the product is so superficial that it is visible it can look blue and will need to be removed.

It is normal for swelling to last up to three weeks after injection so this is not something to plan to do the week before your wedding. Of course the majority of clients have no problems.

Prior to the use of blunt cannuale black eyes were reasonably common results. Unfortunately it is not always possible to use a cannula to do this treatment.

Treating the tear trough decreases the dark circles. As we age it is more common to have a lower eyelid with a distinct border between it and the cheek. This is a good area to treat but it must be treated with caution. Very small amounts are needed in this area. Well done this can make you look years younger.

The aim of treatment is to improve the hollow without interfering with the eye itself. A small amount of filler (<0.5ml) in this area can make a patient look much better. Large amounts are not recommended.

This is not the area for very long lasting fillers as the skin is very thin in this area and any thick filler will be visible. It is going to have to be treated every year.

There is a difference in the placement of fillers under the eyes between those who have had and those who have not had eyelid surgery. Those who have had the fat removed from under their eyes will need to be filled higher up towards the eye. Those with eyebags need to be filled below the eyebag to blend the eyelid into the cheek. This cannot always be made perfect but it can certainly be improved.

For many people the development of an under eye depression coincides with the development of an extended depression into the cheek. We call this the naso-jugal fold. This is the beginning of flattening of the cheek, the first sign that filling of the mid—face will soon be necessary.

NASO LABIAL LINES

These are the lines that run from the end of the nose to the corner of the mouth. They are present even in young people and are often familial. They become deeper with age. Before the advent of deep fillers we treated these lines aggressively but since we have had the thicker deeper fillers to play with emphasis has come off this area somewhat. Removing naso-labial lines completely gives a blank look to the face. If we are going to treat them a great result can be achieved by injecting the area closest to the nose and leaving the rest alone. This avoids giving the face a blank plate like look.

Of course there are certain naso labial lines that need complete filling but It has become obvious since we started filling cheeks and cheekbones that the naso –labial lines were incidentally decreased. If we go back to our table cloth analogy we can see why. The excess tissue from the cheeks is picked up and held up by the filler in the cheeks and therefore does not fold down in the naso—labial area. The naso-labial line is therefore much less obvious and rarely requires filling.

If it is a very deep familial line it is better to attempt to remove it by planning treatment over two sessions as otherwise the filler can be visible.

MARIONETTE LINES

We refer to the lines that go from the corner of the mouth to the jaw as marionette lines. Most often these are folds rather than lines but it can be just lines.

If it is a case of simple lines then a superficial filler will do the job and that is the end of the problem. In this area there can be other problems as well.

When the mouth turns down at the corner we associate this with sadness, so we don't like it. If it is a very minor problem then a filler just in the mouth corner will fix it, end of problem.

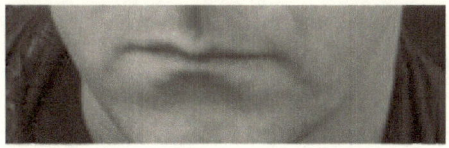

This gentleman is not going to benefit from filler placed in his mouth angles. He has developed a depression that will need to be filled into his chin going towards the jawline. This may be the result of overactivity of muscles or of fat loss.

As we get older the problem becomes more complex. The muscles at the angle of the mouth contribute to the turn down by pulling down excessively. To fix this we inject the aptly named muscle known as the depressor of the angle of the mouth or DAO with muscle relaxant. This allows the mouth to turn up.

The DAO crosses the depressor labii inferioris—the depressor of the lower lip in its lower half. If the depressor labii inferioris is injected instead of the depressor angali ori then the lower lip will be paralysed and will not recover for three months. Make sure your doctor has plenty of experience in injecting this area. That said of course experience has to be gained somewhere.

Muscle relaxant is unlikely to be sufficient for most people. Fillers are also necessary.

Most physicians will do a muscle relaxant injection to the DAO and then ask the patient to come back in two weeks. The reason for this is that the muscle relaxant will change the amount of filler needed in the fold. Before we had muscle relaxants treatment of this area was difficult and expensive for the patient. It was well named the "bottomless pit".

Once again the reason for the difficulty in treating this area was the lack of attention we were paying to the skin laxity above it. It will often be recommended to do this treatment in combination with treating the cheekbones and mid face and using a very thick filler to support the area.

The other problem in this area is the jowl and the pre jowl sulcus. This is the lax area on the jawline that shows as a bulge on the otherwise clear and straight line. This is an absolute giveaway of age. A straight jawline is youthful, one with a bulge is not. To disguise this we use a filler in front of and behind the bulge and sometimes along and behind the jawline itself. This results in a tighter jawline and a decrease in the size of the jowl.

It is important to assess the face prior to doing this because the face shape can be changed positively or negatively. The face can be made broader by injecting along the jaw or the skin tightened by injecting under the jaw. The last thing a broad face needs is to be made broader, but a thin face can benefit from this. This is usually done by cannula injection through a small incision. The use of a cannula is almost essential as damage to the facial artery and serious bruising can happen here.

Muscle relaxant techniques can be used to tighten the jawline but are not always effective and are expensive as a relatively large amount of the product is used. The Thermage technology is also useful here, provided the patient is under sixty and does not have an excessive amount of sagging.

THE NECK

Patients commonly complain that their face is alright, it's just the neck. Face lift surgery also lifts the neck and for some people this is the best answer. For others it is not.

Muscle relaxant injections can decrease the muscle bands that stand out in the neck. As with all other areas this needs to be done three monthly. It is well worth doing. Muscle relaxants can also be injected along the jawline and to the anterior (front) part of the neck. To do this it is a good idea to dilute the product more than usual so that a low dose is given. This will result in a crisper jawline.

If the skin is part of the problem and it almost always is then strengthening the skin will help. Q-Med makes a product called Vital which is perfect for this area. It is injected into the skin all over the neck. This is a very low strength hyaluronic acid product which has been shown to increase the collagen layer in the area. In general this is used in three treatment sessions over three months to great effect. The longevity of this treatment is about twelve months.

The major downside of this treatment is that bruising is almost guaranteed. This is much better done when the weather permits the wearing of a scarf. It is also a treatment that husband and children will be sure to notice. Arrange time off.

Many clients have a red and white speckled appearance on the neck that spares the area under the chin. This is called the Poikiloderma of Civette and is caused by sun exposure. The white area represents the skin shaded from the sun by the chin. It can be easily treated by IPL or laser treatment. Most clients will need two to three treatments maximum. Sunscreen must be used daily to protect the skin. If sunscreen is not used daily then it will recur. Since you now know how important sunscreen is you all use it don't you?

DECOLLETAGE

The neck and décolletage are contiguous and treatment is similar. Muscle relaxants can be used to decrease lines across the chest but most improvement will come from IPL treatment and Vital injections or skin peeling whether chemical or laser.

Pigmentation of the skin is very common in this area and responds well to IPL or laser treatment.

LIPS

As we age our lips lose volume and develop unsightly lines on the top and bottom lip. Lipstick bleeds and becomes an embarrassment. This is much worse if you have the misfortune to lose teeth. The jaw is shrinking and the skin is damaged resulting in the loss of smoothness in the lip and delivering purse string lines around the lip. The result is a lip that is thinner and puckered top and bottom.

Overtreatment of lips is one of the worst results from cosmetic medicine and justifiably it is one of the things most people fear. The time of the trout pout and the duck lip has passed although some still want super large lips. Avoiding trouts and ducks is a matter of injecting the correct area of the lip. When these products were first introduced we were all taught to inject only the outside of the lip producing the duck lip. Then we were taught to inject all across the lip producing a large pneumatic looking lip.

Luckily most doctors have learnt where to place the injections for the best result. It's not just the outline of the lip, nor the entirety of the lip. Best results are achieved by injecting into the natural pillows of the lip. This produces a lovely natural enlargement that is much to be preferred. When there are top and bottom lip lines it is necessary to inject the lines. The aim here is improvement not perfection. Some lines may remain. For older patients there is now a filler that will not enlarge the lips but will fill in the lines in the lip only, giving a fullness but no added bulk to the lips.

It may take some time for some members of the public to warm to the idea that less is more but it is definitely available for those of a more conservative bent. Good lip treatment should be unobtrusive. If this is done well no duckiness will result.

Top and bottom lip lines often need to be injected individually. This is difficult to do without leaving lumps behind. Your doctor may address this by using a cannula to inject above the top and bottom lip or may inject the lines individually. It is a matter of choice. My preference is for a reinforced cannula to the lip line and a sharp needle technique to the lines or cannula again depending on the depth of the lines. The deeper the lines the more likely I am to use a sharp needle and inject the lines directly.

For many clients this is better done in two sessions. This reduces the likelihood of lumps and allows a finer product to be used in layers, but increases the risk of bruising. Bruising is always possible and depends on many things—what is being done, the product and technique used, the supplements the patient is taking, the amount of alcohol the patient drinks. It is not the consequence of poor technique.

Young women want their lips to look full and sexy, they don't always want any change in their shape but sometimes it is necessary. It is certainly possible to give them what they want and not make them look weird. They need their injection into the pillows of the lip top and bottom. The ratio aimed for is top : bottom = 30:70.

It is important to treat the mouth angle in older women often in association with treating the marionette area as described previously. A downward turn to the mouth corner is associated with age. The mouth can easily be turned up or made straight with a filler injected in to the mouth corner with or without muscle relaxant.

Injection of the centre of the lip is rarely a good idea. It makes the lip stick out too far and gives an impression of an overbite. On the other hand, flattening of the frenulum (the depression of the cupid's bow) makes the lip look old and flat. To fix this an injection is placed at the tip of the cupid's bow up to the nose to reinforce the frenulum of the lip but the bow itself is rarely injected. Most injectors will inject from the outer edge to the point of the cupid's bow and not further.

Just remember to leave time between appointments even if you think you want more in your lips. Let it settle for a month and then reassess. It is easy to become addicted to the change and want more and more.

There are clients who push the envelope too far and who want more than is recommended and push the clinician to give them more than enough. These are the ones who end up looking weird. No one wants to create a weird looking face but it happens. Make it a rule. Wait at least a month before having more

Most clients are sensible and understand that perfection is not possible. Great improvement is but it will never be perfect. A face with no movement and absolutely no lines is not attractive and not to be desired.

A face that is well balanced with its good points brought out, major lines removed, lost fat pads replaced and jaw tightened is what we should aim for.

CHIN

Few people think about their chin. We can't see our profile and are not aware it can be improved. It is easy to change the shape of a chin and to make it longer or wider. When people suffer from disproportion of the face adding a few millimetres to the chin can make a huge difference. It is also simple to make the chin come forward to give a more pleasing profile. This can make a pleasant faced girl look beautiful, and an ugly girl look pleasant. A few milimeters are not to be sneezed at.

The thicker fillers are necessary here and will probably be injected over two sessions. Previously to reposition a chin forward required major surgery with cutting and wiring of the jaw. Filling is much more practical. Of course the surgery is forever but the injection takes twenty minutes.

Chins are often irregular and lumpy and heavily creased. This can be fixed by placing a small dose of muscle relaxant in the mentalis muscle correcting the over contraction of muscle insertions in to the skin of the chin. It will also add about one millimetre to the length of the face.

Injecting fillers superficially in this area can be difficult as some clients have very large pores and remnants of old acne that have destroyed the subcutaneous tissue. This results in filler coming out as quickly as it went in. Some improvement is possible doing this but often not sufficient. We need to inject deeply in this area. Multiple product strengths will also be necessary.

SKIN CARE PREPARATIONS THAT WORK

Many people are seduced by the cosmetics industry's glossy advertisements using very beautiful girls assisted by Photoshop as models. People buy the image not the product. The product has no chance of making the purchaser look like the model either before or after Photoshop, because most cosmetics companies spend more money on the promotion, advertising and marketing of their products than they do on the ingredients in side their bottles and jars.

Because we buy the hype and the hope the packaging and advertising are very important. Most cosmetic brands started out with a single person making up a 'miracle "cream at home and selling from there. Few, if any started in a high tech laboratory.

It should come as no surprise that the vast majority of cosmetics purchased at great cost have no hope of producing any change in the skin. The surprising thing is that purchasers do not return the products and complain of the lack of efficacy. Subconsciously I guess we don't expect them to work.

The introduction of cosmeceuticals has changed that. Cosmeceuticals are not generally available in department stores or beauty therapy salons. The strength of the products makes it unfeasible for them to be sold by unqualified people. You may find some with limited efficacy there but not the more effective ones. These you will only find in high end day spas associated with doctors.

Our TPG (therapeutic goods administration) the equivalent of the US FDA has very stringent rules for cosmetics and consistently removes effective products from preparations. The cosmeceutical industry is kept busy finding the derivatives of the product no longer approved. It is a game where the manufacturers and constantly finding derivatives that are more active than the banned parent compound. No one objects to this if the complaint is that the product is harmful, but if it is done to make sure a product doesn't work and can therefore be classified as a cosmetic it is very annoying.

These products are effective and potent and need to be prescribed correctly and for that reason should not be sold or purchased on the internet. I will not rely on the strength of a product bought on the internet and will not increase the strength of my own treatments when a patient has been using internet bought products, no matter what it says on the jar. I need to know what my patient has been using.

Most anti-ageing products contain alpha hydroxy acids in a wash, retinol or its derivatives as a serum, vitamin C, B and E, plus or minus other anti-oxidants, peptides, metalo—matrix protease inhibitors, and growth factors.

Lactic acid plus vitamin A,C,E and B and sunscreen is the most common prescription for sun related ageing changes.

In this country there are two very inexpensive and well known ranges using these ingredients,

ASAP and Aspect, that are available readily. These products are very inexpensive. The doctor only variant is Aspect Dr. It is a much better formulated product and causes less irritation. ASAP is suitable mainly for acne as it is a little drying for those concerned with ageing and sun related damage.

It is impossible to give a relevant exhaustive list of active products but the following are the most reliable I have been able to find.

Skinstitute	low cost basic range. Active
Restylane	Low cost, minimal activity but a good night serum.
Ultraceuticals	High cost basic active range
Aspect Doctor	Low cost basic and beyond (incorporates good products for Rosacea)
PCA	Moderate price. Full range not available in Australia. Good Vitamin A and C products
Cosmedix	Moderate price. Very active but limited range of product.
Results Rx	High price. Excellent products, very active—may need to start with a less active range first.
Skin Medica	High tech. Products are very active, contain peptides and growth factors. Excellent products.
Societe	Moderate—high price. Contains peptides mimicking viper venom for line relaxation. Highly active products.
AgeLOC	Moderate—high price. The first genetic modulator on the market. This product differs from all the others by being effective at the genetic level. It causes rejuvenation of the cellular processes in the cells by bio effective stimulation. In other words it makes your skin cells behave as if they were younger. Excellent product. No competitor.

Most people have products that they love that have no active ingredients in them. For some they love the fact that these are organic, or prepared locally, or they love the fragrance or the feel on the skin.

Regular maintenance with these sorts of products will not renew the skin in any way but regular beautician treatment with massage and masks will help. Some beautician ranges are moderately active against acne and blackheads and others for sensitive skins are calming but they do not treat the cause and signs of ageing.

As always, a girl's best friend is her sunscreen. In this country it should be worn daily, summer and winter, on the face, neck (Including the back) décolletage, hands, arms and legs if they are not covered.

Skin cancers occur commonly on the face, particularly on the nose, brow ridges, sides of the cheeks, neck, scalp, legs and feet. Melanoma can be anywhere but, in women, it is commonly found on the calf and back of the upper arm. Women are not the only ones who need to use sunscreen. Children need to be protected too. Mothers tend to protect their children well but forget about themselves. Men in this country consider a dab of zinc on the nose is the only protection they need for a day's golf. Very few treat their skin actively. At best they borrow a dab of cream from their partner if their skin feels a bit tight. The incidence of skin cancer is much higher in men than in women and it is no wonder.

Some men are now starting to use cosmetics and some ranges are targeted directly at men. Because this is an area of new expenditure for men they do not start straight away with active products, rather they buy something from the supermarket or the chemist. As they become more sophisticated in this area they will be more willing to spend on the products they need to protect themselves.

It is often said that men do not age as quickly as women because they shave every day and exercise the face as they do it. There is a lot of truth in this, not because of the exercise but because when they shave they are exfoliating the skin and causing micro trauma. The response of the skin to exfoliation and micro trauma is to thicken up and renew.

This is what we are going to talk about now.

LIGHTS, BURNS, PEELS AND TRAUMA

Before Cleopatra took her baths in fermented mare's milk (alpha hydroxyl acid) the Persians were using fire to treat and remove wrinkles. A light burn to the skin will cause the skin to tighten and lessen wrinkles but imagine the result if the physician got it wrong and left the fire a little too long! Whilst this is earliest approximation of laser treatment it is uncontrolled and not to be tried at home.

If we are trying to get the skin to increase its turnover of cells to produce fresh, young looking skin we need to do it safely. Many types of skin wounding have been tried. All will be effective to some degree.

Skin needling Initially this was done around the eyes with or without the injection of any substance and line reduction happened. The modern equivalent of this is the roller with fine needles attached. It is rolled over the skin to produce micro wounds which heal instantly and result in tightening of the skin and increased cell turnover.

The needles on these rollers vary in length and vary in efficacy. The fine, short needles do not hurt, but the longer ones do. The shorter ones can be used at home. Depending on skin type

(colour) it may be necessary to prepare the skin with pigment controlling products.

This treatment is effective for acne scarring as well as sun damage. Results will vary and take up to six months. Most clients will have in clinic treatment monthly and continue their treatment at home with a shorter roller. With continued treatment very good results can be expected. Treatment will continue for three to six months.

This is the least expensive type of physical skin rejuvenation. It is useful for treating wrinkles and acne scars. Good skin care is essential with this. It is not a particularly painful treatment but you do need to do it to yourself at home as well as have clinic treatment.

MICRODERMABRASION

Good results occur from micro dermabrasion on fine acne scars and fine wrinkles. It is mainly used to help remove blackheads and whiteheads and to stimulate the skin to repair and replace dead cells. For clients with good skin microdermabrasion makes the skin glow. For clients with minor acne it decreases pore blockage by removing dead cells. It is usually done monthly in clinic and combined with active skin care products.

It is unlikely to change anything but the finest scars and wrinkles but it will improve the condition of the skin and make it much healthier.

DERMABRASION

This procedure is still done but not as frequently as it used to be. It can be used to treat severe acne scarring and deep wrinkles and is not for the faint hearted. It is usually performed under general anaesthetic and requires a ten day recovery period. The skin is taken down to the level where it bleeds. Healing comes from the cells in the sebaceous glands and will take up to ten days. Expect to be at home with a very uncomfortable face for at least a week.

LASERS

Dermabrasion has largely been replaced by Fractional laser treatment. Sometimes it is still used to treat top lip lines but it can result in depigmentation if done too aggressively. Fraxel is a brand name for Co2 fractional laser. There are many fractional lasers with similar effects. Naturally the distributors protect their brand name and object to its being used to describe other lasers.

Lasers are often misunderstood by the general public and also by some beauty therapists who use them.

Lasers produce a single colour of light with the light beams all being synchronous. The beam does not diverge and is very strong. The light travels in a straight line without splaying out. Light is the result of electrical stimulation of a certain gas with electrons being accelerated in the laser chamber and being enhanced by reflection in the chamber. The light escapes through a pin hole and therefore only light waves going in the one direction can get out. Diode lasers produce a pure coloured light but do not have a tube. The light is produced by electrical manipulation. These are much more reliable than lasers that depend on a tube. In past years lasers were more likely to be lying on the floor in pieces than actually operating.

IPL or intense pulsed light is a different thing all together. The light from IPL is not all going in one direction and is not in phase. This means that it is not as strong as laser light.

There are many things that can be changed in settings on lasers and IPLs to get the desired effect but only if the machine can produce the wavelength of light that is required. Unfortunately not every laser treats every problem. If laser power, pulse duration, spot size and inter pulse distance can't be changed then it is going to be of limited usefulness. These are things for the operator to determine. From the consumer's point of view the laser has to be suitable for the treatment prescribed.

The skin colour of the patient is important: darker skinned patients suffer more complications from laser and IPL treatments than fair skinned patients. The commonest problem after laser treatment is inflammatory increase in pigment. Light skinned patients are unlikely to get this but are advised to avoid sun for a few weeks after treatment. Dark skinned patients, particularly skin types V and VI (dark Indian and Negro) are better treated on some lasers than others and should be treated with creams that reduce the production of melanin for at least four weeks before treatment.

Lasers are selected to treat a specific target tissue, whether it is hair, pigment or water.

Fraxel is a fractional Co2 laser. The light it produces is absorbed by water. As our skin is full of water it is very effective on the skin. The laser can be used in two ways—to remove all the skin or just remove spots of it. This is used to remove acne scars, wrinkle and pigment spots.

Complete removal or ablation of the skin will produce a much better result for most people but will require ten days downtime and be an unpleasant experience. This is why most people choose to have what is called a "non ablative "treatment. It only drills little holes. These little holes heal almost immediately. The treatment makes the skin dark for a week, then it peels.

Saying a laser is fractional means that it has a head that treats areas spot by spot and spares the skin between the spots. This allows the skin to recover quickly. As most of the skin is spared in this sort of treatment the treatment needs to be repeated. Significant improvement will occur with one treatment but further improvement will occur by repeating the treatment.

This type of laser is used for treating acne scarring and for skin rejuvenation. There will be a darkening of the skin over five days and then the dark skin will peel off leaving fresh skin beneath. Wrinkles will be improved by fractional laser treatment but the best effect is always from a full ablative treatment. This leaves the skin red raw for up to ten days. Most people choose to do a fractional treatment with the lower downtime but the result from ablative treatment is superior.

Fractional CO_2 treatment laser is also very effective for removing pigmentation. It can be used on darker skin but post inflammatory pigmentation (increased pigmentation) can occur even if the patient is pretreated with anti pigmentation products. This increase in pigment will go away but it is a trying period for patient and physician. Sun avoidance and sun screen are also very important in the treatment of all types of pigmentation.

Most clients with acne scarring will require more than one treatment. The average number of treatments for severe acne scarring is four.

Treatment for pigmentation will usually require multiple treatments too as well as a rigid cosmetic treatment plan and obsessive protection for the sun.

Lasers for hair removal target the bulb of the hair deep in the dermis. The latest for this is the 808nm laser which claims to remove blonde and white hair as well as dark hair. The NdYag laser at 1064nm is excellent for hair removal on dark skinned clients. Most problems with hair removal occur because of choosing the wrong machine for the client's skin type. Most of my patients have skin type 2 and 3. Recent immigration form South America has brought a significant number of type 4 patients as well.

My choice of hair removal laser is simple because skin type is rarely an issue. My main concerns are the speed of operation and the technology surrounding the cooling of the tip. Contrary to most people's expectation lasers applied to the skin hurt. Technology to cool the skin down during treatment determines the amount of discomfort felt.

Newer machines have built in cooling systems that cool the tip that touches the skin decreasing pain a lot. Some machines will rely on the simultaneous use of a Zimmer cooler to make the treatment less unpleasant.

The size of the treatment head is important to me but probably not for you. It helps make the treatment faster.

The speed of the machine is also dependent on the ability of the machine to fire at the same power repeatedly. Most machines lose power and need a rest after an hour or two—just like us.

I rely on the Fitzpatrick skin type system which follows.

Very fair—	never tan always burn	=type 1
Fair	usually burns may tan	= type 2
Darker	tans doesn't burn	= type 3
Dark Italian	/ Greek never burns	= type 4
Indian dark		= type 5
Negro		= type 6

Those with skin types 4, 5, and 6 should take great care.

Until the last twenty years our population was overwhelmingly type 1, 2 and some type 3 skins. Now 3, 4,5, and six are much more common. Darker skins often pigment following laser or other treatment. Clinicians will be more cautious treating them. Most will insist on pre treatment skin products and test areas. This is very sensible.

Removing tattoos requires a laser light that will be absorbed by the different colours in the tattoo. As tattoos contain black, red, green and sometimes other colours it can be a long term treatment as the colours are usually removed one at a time. Clients always complain that it costs more to have that tattoo removed than it did to have it put on in the first place. A plain black tattoo is the easiest to remove. The tattoos often leave a ghost outline behind, so our treatments are not perfect.

Cosmetic tattoos can be an issue when treating with Thermage a radio frequency treatment. The treatment can turn cosmetic tattoos black. All operators should be aware of this and avoid treating directly over cosmetic tattoos.

Vascular lasers target haemoglobin and close down blood vessels by creating a thermal shock wave inside the vessel. This results in injury to the vessel wall. Natural repair processes then close the vessel down so that no blood flows through it and the vessel disappears. The depth of the blood vessels in the skin is important. Some lasers are effective on the face but not on the larger, deeper vessels in the legs because the laser light varies in its penetration. Many doctors still treat small and large veins in the legs by injecting substances that will cause local injury in the blood vessel. The body then blocks these vessels off in the same way as it repairs the damage. This is called sclerotherapy. There are a number of different drugs that can be used for this. Naturally their availability will vary from country to country. The commonest drug used here is polidocanol.

The newest vein treatment is treatment of varicose veins by feeding a laser fibre into the vein after pin pointing the area of disease by prior ultrasound. The laser is then fired at the problem area. This is called endovascular laser treatment and is very effective in the treatment of varicose veins decreasing the need for surgery. It is a walk in walk out procedure one under local anaesthetic and does not require hospital admission.

RADIO FREQUENCY DEVICES THERMAGE AND ULTHERA

All treatments aiming to tighten skin or make skin fresher first cause damage in the skin. The natural repair mechanisms of the body then increase collagen production and skin tightening and stimulate skin cell turnover. This is true of Co2 laser, all radio frequency devices, dermabrasion (micro or macro), skin needling and injections of stimulant proteins. Low powered laser applications do not damage they simply stimulate but the results are less visible.

Radio frequency either mono polar or bipolar focuses radio waves under the skin. This heats the existing collagen til it shrinks and stimulates more collagen growth in the shrunken tissue. Think of it as gathering stitch followed by a tacking stitch. There is an immediate tightening followed by further growth of new collagen over a six month period.

If the correct patient is chosen for this treatment the results can be very good. However if the client has lost too much tightness in the skin then the results can be very disappointing. This is most suitable for younger clients in their late thirties through to fifties.

The procedure takes approximately an hour. It is definitely an uncomfortable procedure but no discomfort is felt after treatment. The skin may be a little pink after treatment but otherwise it leaves no evidence behind. The changes are subtle but worthwhile if the patient is in the correct age group. This does not mean to say that older patients cannot have treatment. Some get very good results but it is less reliable than with younger clients.

Treatment should not be repeated at less than six month intervals because the new collagen that has been stimulated to grow will be destroyed just as it is produced.

IPL

Intense pulsed light is not the same as Laser. The light produced is of multiple wavelengths and is filtered to achieve the correct wavelength. This means that it is not as strong. IPL is very effective for removing small blood vessels, removing brown spots and some pigmentation and stimulating collagen production.

The same precautions apply to ILP as to laser with regard to skin type and to the need to be able to manipulate the pulse duration and inter pulse distance.

IPL teatments can be enhanced by using them after microdermabrasion or skin needling.

The stimulation is similar but stronger than that provided by lower powered devices like **Omnilux**. Naturally some people get better results from this type of collagen stimulation than others. This is a safe treatment with virtually no downside.

Omnilux can also be used to activate drugs for the treatment of basal cell skin cancers (BCCs). Unless the cancer is aggressive or in an area that is prone to recurrence this is a very good method of treatment. Unfortunately the appropriate drug is expensive and it is not universally subsidised in my country. Perhaps it will be soon.

A lower strength of the same drug can be used to produce a peel of the facial skin. This will also remove precancerous skin lesions. This treatment can result in a lot of swelling of the face and because the drug used makes the skin sun and light sensitive for seventy two hours after application hiding in the dark at home is an absolute necessity. The result will be beautiful skin without pigmentation or redness but if you live in a house with huge windows that let in the sun all day you will find it difficult to find somewhere to hide.

CONCLUSION

This is not meant to be an exhaustive study of every method used for facial rejuvenation, just a brief guide to what can be done without surgery.

Facial treatment can be divided in to the need for muscle relaxation and structural problems. My opinion has always been that the lines on a face are not as ageing as lack of adequate support for the skin.

If a client has good cheekbones and a strong chin she will maintain her looks much longer than the one who has little support in the cheek and has always had a flat face.

The search for the way to keep all lines at bay is in my opinion misdirected. If we can keep the structural supports and the crisp lines of the jaw strong then we will look young despite some lines. Flat immobile faces are not my ideal of beauty.

The quality of the skin is a major component of youth and beauty. I believe that a face with no lines but with large pores, irregular pigmentation and scaly patches of sun damage is not attractive and not youthful. Those who treat only their facial lines are not treating themselves as well as possible.

The question for you, the reader, is to decide what should be done. No one should think that by employing these techniques that age can be kept at bay completely and that we will all look forever twenty. The most sensible approach is to keep oneself looking your best at whatever age. Nothing is worse than overdone rejuvenation. This is an art more than a science and one of the main attributes of the artist is to know when enough is enough.

Trust your treating physician. Don't try for perfect. Settle for looking great!

www.ingramcontent.com/pod-product-compliance
Lightning Source LLC
Chambersburg PA
CBHW022132170526
45157CB00004B/1844